# Reality Activities

## A How To Manual
## for Increasing Orientation

### Second Edition

Richelle N. Cunninghis, Ed.M. OTR/L

## Idyll Arbor, Inc.

PO Box 720, Ravensdale, WA 98051 (206) 432-3231

ISBN 1-882883-21-7

# Table of Contents

**Publisher's Note:**

We have promoted the development and publishing of this book because we feel that those who receive the services of a therapist or activity professional deserve the best possible care. This book was written for licensed, certified or registered therapists and certified activity directors (or those studying to become such).

To the best of our knowledge, the information and recommendations of this book reflect currently accepted practice. Nevertheless, they can not be considered absolute and universal. Recommendations for activities for a particular individual must be considered in light of the individual's needs and condition. The authors and publisher disclaim responsibly for any adverse effects resulting directly or indirectly from the suggested activities, from any undetected errors or from the reader's misunderstanding of the text.

**Acknowledgments**

Cover photograph by Spirit Wind, Kent, WA.

The art work contained in this book was obtained from Corel Gallery (Corel Corporation, P.O. Box 3595, Salinas, CA 93912-3595) and The Print Shop® Deluxe (Brøderbund Software, Inc., 500 Redwood Blvd., Novato, CA 94948-6121).

# Introduction

Being oriented to "reality" is knowing who one is, where one is, when it is and what the key objects around one are. As some people age they may lose some mental sharpness. This loss is frequently caused by the slow deterioration of the brain (dementia). Injuries which cause damage to the brain such as strokes and head injuries may also decrease a person's orientation to reality. This loss may or may not be

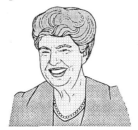

permanent depending on the reason for the loss and the amount of mental exercise the person engages in. The time of the day and the amount of energy a person has also makes a difference in his/her ability to remain oriented. A common effect of a loss of orientation is "sun downing" which is the loss of orientation as the day draws to an end.

Reality orientation and other similar techniques have long been accepted as effective tools in the management of those who are confused and disoriented. Much has been written and many training programs have been presented on the philosophy, rationale and procedures for using these techniques. But little seems to be available on implementation — how materials and activities can best be used for the practical application of the principles.

Experience has shown that boredom and monotony have caused the failure of many of these programs. Personnel have reported that they feel a lack of spontaneity and originality in their programming and that this often gets transmitted to the participants themselves.

The purpose of this book is to provide practical suggestions and lists of ideas for reality activities; they have been gathered from many different sources in an attempt to show the great range of possibilities. No theory or background information is included except where it relates to the activities being described.

Designed as a guide for those working with persons with all levels of disorientation — slight to severe — the book offers instructions on how activities can be adapted to meet needs at any level. Try the activities in this book. You will find that working with these residents is easier. A companion book, **Activities for the Elderly Volume 2** by Parker and Will[1] gives you 80 more activities to use with residents who have problems with reality orientation.

# Task Breakdown

One of the most important secrets of running a successful reality orientation program is knowing how to break activities down into smaller steps. Each step is called a task. The purpose of task breakdown is to involve residents at a level which they are capable of doing. To begin, residents do steps which they are able to do. Eventually, they may be able to complete the whole activity.

The activity may be as simple as opening a door to go into the next room or as complex as making a three course dinner from scratch. This chapter will show you how to break down activities into numerous tasks and to identify which tasks are easier then others.

The easiest way to break any activity into tasks is to do the activity yourself, slowly. As you make each movement, ask yourself four questions:

1.  What did I have to know to make this move? (cognitive)
2.  What set of muscles did I need to use and/or coordinate? (physical)
3.  How and with whom did I need to interact? (social)
4.  How did it make me feel? (emotional)

Although the cognitive, physical and social components are fairly easy to identify for any given activity, the emotional component is often somewhat more difficult. This refers to the feelings that the activity triggers, not only in the doing, but in the anticipating and remembering, as well. These may be very different for each person, according to his/her past experience and individual value system, and may include such things as nostalgia, pleasure, anxiety, memory enhancement, increased self-esteem, success or embarrassment.[2]

Moreover, there are a range of emotional reactions that might be expected for a particular activity and these should be listed as part of the task breakdown.

To see how a task breakdown can be done, imagine yourself sitting in a circle with ten other people, each one of you facing into the center of the circle. The person three to your right has a colorful beach ball which she seems to be passing to the other people on your right. To break down this activity into tasks, imagine what you would do step by step. First you would look to your right. You need to realize that the ball is coming toward you. You have a sense that you are to copy the actions of those before you by taking the ball from the person on your right and then passing it to the person on your left. Next you would wait for the ball to come back to you. The next three pages show the task breakdown for the beach ball activity.

# Passing the Beach Ball

**You need to realize that the ball is coming toward you.**

1. What did I have to know to make this move? (cognitive)
   I would need to:
   - realize that the ball is coming toward me.
   - recognize a pattern (passing to the left).

2. What set of muscles did I need to use and/or coordinate? (physical)
   I would need to:
   - turn my head to the right.
   - watch with my eyes the ball being passed.

3. How and with whom did I need to interact? (social)
   I would need to:
   - wait for the ball to come to me so that I was not distracted or distracting others.

4. What is the appropriate emotional response for this movement? (emotional)
   I would need to:
   - display a neutral to mildly excited emotional response, or
   - show some irritation or embarrassment at choice of activity (due to perceived age inappropriateness, perceived skill level, etc.) or
   - exhibit some signs of anxiety (fear of not performing adequately, being judged by peers, etc.).

**You have a sense that you are to copy the actions of those before you by taking the ball from the person on your right and then passing it to the person on your left.**

1. What did I have to know to make this move? (cognitive)
   I would need to:
   - know to reach for a ball.
   - know the correct amount of pressure to put on the sides of the ball so that it does not drop or go shooting out of my hands.
   - know that I was to pass the ball on to the person next to me on my left.

2. What set of muscles did I need to use and/or coordinate? (physical)
   I would need to:
   - have eye-hand coordination to grasp the ball.
   - have the ability to hold the ball as I moved it across the midline of my body to my left side.
   - be able to control the speed of my movements.

3. How and with whom did I need to interact? (social)
   I would need to:
   - make visual contact with the people on my right and left (but not necessarily eye to eye).
   - cooperate with the people on my right and left for a safe transfer of the ball (without dropping it).

4. What is the appropriate emotional response for this movement? (emotional)
   I would need to:
   - display a neutral to mildly excited emotional response, or

- show some irritation or embarrassment at choice of activity (due to perceived age inappropriateness, perceived skill level, etc.) or
- exhibit some signs of anxiety (fear of not performing adequately, being judged by peers, etc.).

**Next you would wait for the ball to come back to you**

1. What did I have to know to make this move? (cognitive)
   I would need to:
   - know how to wait.

2. What set of muscles did I need to use and/or coordinate? (physical)
   I would need to:
   - be able to stay seated in my chair without falling.
   - be able to stay in my chair without excessive body movements.

3. How and with whom did I need to interact? (social)
   I would need to:
   - limit my social interactions to ones that would not interfere with the reasonable movement of the ball around the circle.

4. What is the appropriate emotional response for this movement? (emotional)
   I would need to:
   - display a neutral to mildly excited emotional response, or
   - show some irritation or embarrassment at choice of activity (due to perceived age inappropriateness, perceived skill level, etc.) or
   - exhibit some signs of anxiety (fear of not performing adequately, being judged by peers, etc.).

Breaking activities down into smaller tasks is easy if you go slowly, think about what you are doing as you do it and write your actions (and thoughts and emotions) down. Many professionals find it easier to modify activities for residents if they place all cognitive skills together, as well as all physical, social and emotional skills together. This way the list can be used like a check list; checking "yes" if the resident can do the task and checking "no" if s/he cannot.

The chart on the next page shows you the task breakdown we just did but this time it is written like a checklist assessment form. If you already know that your resident cannot use his right arm because of a stroke, you can modify the activity before you start. By looking at the list of tasks under "physical" you will find only one or two tasks that may need some modification. If your resident has a short attention span you will find only three or four tasks that may require some verbal cues from you for the resident to successfully complete the activity.

**Task Breakdown: Passing a Beach Ball**

| Cognitive | Yes | No | Comments |
|---|---|---|---|
| realize that the ball is coming | | | |
| recognize a pattern (passing to the left) | | | |
| know to reach for a ball | | | |
| know the correct amount of pressure to put on the sides of the ball so that it does not drop or go shooting out of hands | | | |
| know to pass the ball on to the person next to left | | | |
| know how to wait | | | |
| **Physical** | **Yes** | **No** | **Comments** |
| turn head to the right (then left) | | | |
| watch the ball being passed | | | |
| adequate eye-hand coordination to grasp the ball | | | |
| hold the ball as it is moved across midline from right to left | | | |
| control the speed of movements | | | |
| stay seated in chair without falling | | | |
| stay in chair without excessive body movements | | | |
| **Social** | **Yes** | **No** | **Comments** |
| wait for the ball to come so not be distracted or to distract others | | | |
| make visual contact with the person on right then left (but not necessarily eye to eye visual contact) | | | |
| cooperate with the person on right then on left to allow a safe transfer of the ball (so that it does not drop) | | | |
| limit social interactions to those that would not interfere with the reasonable movement of the ball around the circle | | | |
| **Emotional** | **Yes** | **No** | **Comments** |
| display emotional response within expected range | | | |

By looking at all of the tasks required (the whole picture) you will be better able to know exactly what the resident is able to do on any given day. Residents tend to have "good" and "bad" days. On good days s/he may be able to complete 70% of all the task for passing the beach ball. But what if you notice that the resident is less and less able to cross midline? This information will be very important to share with the other team members as you help identify the residents strengths and needs.

When a resident is not able to complete an activity successfully you may still find that s/he can do some or most of the tasks which make up that activity. By breaking the activity down into task units you will be able to help the resident with only those tasks that s/he needs help. When you help the resident with only those parts (tasks) of the activity which s/he can't do independently and allowing him/her to do those which s/he can, you help empower the resident.

Residents who have problems with orientation will tend to retain, at least for a while, cognitive knowledge and skills learned earlier in life. It is normal for residents with dementia to lose newly learned information first. The physical movements and coordination learned through repeated involvement in an activity in the past tends to stay with the resident longer then the cognitive knowledge and skills. When selecting activities look for those activities that have strong roots in physical movements the resident has done for decades. This movement will tend to stimulate the resident's greatest potential for cognitive orientation.

Some tasks are harder then others. Threading a needle is more difficult then passing a rope through a large hoop. Three elements determine how difficult a task is:

1. degree of control required (coordination and self monitoring)
2. degree of training required (knowledge and skill)
3. number of multiple tasks required to be completed at one time (monitoring numerous events at one time, using judgment to modify performance and understanding how each of the tasks affects the other)

A task is "simple" if a typical adult would find the task non-stressful, easy to perform and/or did not involve more then one or two actions for any one task. Opening a door, stating one's name, sorting obviously different types of items into two piles, moving a checker piece on a board or greeting another person would be simple tasks.

A task is "moderately difficult" if a typical adult would find the task requires some thought, purposeful coordination of one's body and/or involved two to three actions in a relatively short time span. Reading the newspaper, completing a pencil and paper maze, using a walker and dancing with a partner at the same time, painting a still life, discussing Dear Abby's advice with two other people and sorting similar objects into different piles would all be moderately difficult tasks.

A task has "greater complexity" if a typical adult would find the task requires thought and concentration, a degree of physical coordination that comes only with serious practice, and/or involves three or more actions in a relatively short time span. Working on cross stitch, writing a journal, driving a scooter, cooking a meal from scratch and problem solving a conflict with a friend would all be complex tasks.

Passing the beach ball is a relatively simple task. Only moderate physical control is required, little training is necessary to pass a ball while sitting and only one major task is required at a time to be successful.

Once you break your activities down into specific tasks and decide how difficult each task is, you will be able to better decide which residents would benefit the most from different activities. By inviting residents of similar ability levels to appropriate activities you may decrease agitation (frustration) and increase self esteem.

On the next page you will find one activity (The Food Game) which has different tasks listed along with a suggested degree of difficulty. You can use this as a guide as you evaluate your own activities. Following the Food Game is a blank task checklist chart for you to use as you break down your activities into separate tasks.

# The Food Game[3]

To set up this game, the staff cuts out pictures of fruit from magazines, glues the pictures of each kind of fruit onto its own piece of white typing paper, writes the name of the fruit in large letters (at least 2 inches tall) on the paper and then laminates each paper. The card for "cherries" would have pictures of cherries and the word *cherry* written out on the card. The resident is to sort empty food containers onto the appropriate fruit card. For the word "cherry" the staff may have a box of cherry Jell-O, a box of cherry flavored cake and a can of cherries. Depending in the severity of dementia, the staff may use just one, two or more fruit cards.

- Apples: applesauce, apple strudel, apple pie, apple juice, baked apples, Applette candy bar.
- Pears: pear nectar, canned pears
- Grapes: wine, grape juice, raisins, grape jelly, grape chewing gum.
- Oranges: orange juice, orange marmalade, orange Jell-O, orange cake mix.
- Bananas: banana cream pie, banana cake, banana muffins, banana nut bread.
- Cherries: cherry Jell-O, cherry cookies, maraschino cherries, cherry cough drops, cherry pie.

1. Identify types of food on laminated cards. (*simple; moderate*)
2. Identify types of food on empty packages. (*simple; moderate*)
3. Demonstrates ability to match pictures on paper with pictures/names on empty packages. (*greater complexity*)
4. Demonstrates ability to sort empty packages between two different kinds of fruit. (*greater complexity*)
5. Demonstrates ability to sort empty packages between three (or more) different kinds of fruit. (*greater complexity*)

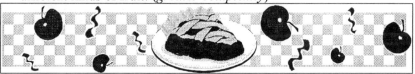

**Task:**

| Cognitive | Yes | No | Comments |
|---|---|---|---|
|  |  |  |  |
|  |  |  |  |
|  |  |  |  |
|  |  |  |  |
|  |  |  |  |
|  |  |  |  |
| **Physical** | Yes | No | Comments |
|  |  |  |  |
|  |  |  |  |
|  |  |  |  |
|  |  |  |  |
|  |  |  |  |
|  |  |  |  |
| **Social** | Yes | No | Comments |
|  |  |  |  |
|  |  |  |  |
|  |  |  |  |
|  |  |  |  |
|  |  |  |  |
| **Emotional** | Yes | No | Comments |
|  |  |  |  |
|  |  |  |  |

# Sorting Activities

For individuals who are confused and have short attention spans, one of the simplest tasks involves selecting or sorting. Beads, shells, yarns, buttons or anything of differing colors and/or shapes may be used.

It is best to start by having the resident pick out "all the blue ones" or "all the round ones that look like this." This is far less overwhelming than asking the resident to sort them all. After selecting by color, they might be sorted by size or shape, picking one characteristic at a time.

This can also be done with a deck of playing cards — first the red ones are selected, then the hearts. The process may be continued by asking the resident to indicate which card of a pair is higher. A natural progression may lead to a game of War, where the resident would have to recognize the higher card. From this point, the resident may be able to count the cards, determine who has won and, possibly even move on to other card games.

The concept that is described here can be used with almost any activity and is an illustration of task breakdown. The materials are introduced in a simple, repetitive way. Once the individual is familiar with them, s/he is asked to add another step, still using the same basic materials.

The resident will be able to perform better if you select activities s/he has done for a long time. The table on the next pages gives you some ideas.

# Everyday Sorting Activities

| Object | Sorting Activity |
|---|---|
| **silver ware/flat ware** | • by type (spoon, fork, knife)<br>• by setting (one knife, fork, spoon)<br>• by pattern |
| **socks** | • by pairs<br>• by color<br>• by size |
| **coins** | • by type (penny, nickel, dime)<br>• by amount (25¢, $1.00)<br>• by size |
| **groceries** | • by food type (vegetable, fruit)<br>• by container type (box, can, jar)<br>• by meals (combine to make a meal)<br>• by cost (under $1.00, over $2.00) |
| **nuts and bolts** | • by type (nuts, bolts, screws, washers)<br>• by pairs (that fit together)<br>• by metal type (brass, steel) |
| **keys and locks** | • match keys to locks<br>• match locks by type (combination, key)<br>• by brand |
| **mail**<br>**(laminate envelopes)** | • by type (bills, letters, junk)<br>• by who they are addressed to<br>• by address<br>• by size |

| Object | Sorting Activity |
|---|---|
| **comic strips**<br>**(glued on heavier paper then**<br>**laminated)** | • by comic strip<br>• by order of story<br>• by story line (short humor,<br>ongoing story) |
| **salt and pepper shakers** | • by salt and by pepper<br>• by matching paired containers |
| **writing utensils** | • by type (pen, pencil, magic<br>marker, crayon)<br>• by color |
| **keys** | • by type (car, house)<br>• by size |
| **thread** | • by color (blues, greens, reds,<br>yellows)<br>• by brand names<br>• by thickness |
| **recipe cards**<br>**(laminate cards)** | • by food type (main course,<br>salad)<br>• by ingredients (meats, fruit)<br>• by whole meal (plan complete<br>meal) |
| **handbells** | • by size<br>• by tone<br>• by scale (do, re, me, fa, so, la,<br>ti, do) |
| **office supplies** | • by type (rubber band, paper<br>clips) |
| **seed packets** | • by type (flowers, vegetables)<br>• by plant (tomatoes, sunflowers) |

# Matching Activities

Matching activities, too, are particularly suitable for residents who are confused and the choices of materials are, practically speaking, limitless.

One technique involves cutting pairs of the same shape out of a variety of different textures, such as sandpaper, velvet, fur, leather, satin, tissue paper, etc. The resident is given one of a pair and asked to find its match **by feel only.** Again, in the beginning the resident might be offered only two or three choices (in a paper bag or with his/her eyes closed). Each time the resident has selected successfully a few more items could be added.

Instead of touch, one of the other senses might be employed in the same type of activity — **matching similar odors, shapes, colors or sounds** — always beginning with limited choices which can be increased both in number and in difficulty as success is attained.

**Melody bells** (small hand bells which are made true to pitch and cover a complete musical scale) are especially nice to have on hand to use with your residents. The resident can try to match pitch.

**Pictures** are another vehicle for matching activities. Cut-outs from magazines can be utilized in a variety of activities, including selecting:

— the two which are the same (in the beginning
providing one and asking the resident to match
it from a very limited number of choices)
— a "little one" which is like a "big one"
— colors ("can you find another red one?")
— similar objects (such as
cats, cars, flowers, etc.—
the pictures not being
identical but depicting
the same type of thing)
— go-together (bread and
butter, Blondie and
Dagwood, boat and oars)
— pictures which match
actual objects (This is
often difficult for people who are confused to
do.)

Again, these activities are graded as to difficulty, simple
matching being the least complex. It is helpful to keep a file
of suitable pictures, mounting them on index cards and
laminating them for durability, ease of handling, ease of
cleaning and lessened confusion because they will all be the
same size and shape. If you are able to use pictures larger
than the standard 3" x 5", the residents will be able to see
them better.

**Name recognition** also lends itself to matching activities in a
variety of ways. Since recognition of self and others is one
of the prime aims of reality activities, it is good practice to
incorporate name recognition activities frequently. One
possible approach is to print the resident's name on a board
or paper, provide letters (wood, felt, plastic are possibilities)
and ask the resident to select the appropriate letters. Many
people who cannot write or spell their names can do this

successfully. (You may need to start with the simpler task of letter recognition first.) The resident might also be asked to select his own from several name tags that are offered. The next steps might be to recognize his/her written name after having only heard it spoken, to repeat other people's names in the group, to spell out other people's names and to be able to distribute the appropriate name tags to others in the group.

Reality information can also be presented through such matching activities as the:

— **date** (duplicating what is on the appropriate line of the reality orientation board)
— **time** (making the hands on the clock match those of the one on the wall)
— **place** (picking out the appropriate one from selections offered)

The more that you are able to use every day objects in your matching, the better your residents will be able to do. Use your imagination!

# *Real Life Props*

It is desirable to use real objects whenever possible as their use reduces the confusion factor. And, although participants may exhibit signs of confusion, it is important to remember that they are adults and may be offended at the use of certain childish materials. (This, of course, depends on how they are presented and how they are utilized.) In addition there is often not much money available and the use of everyday, common, readily obtainable items helps keep costs down. The range of suitable materials is almost endless and only limited by one's own imagination.

Orientation to time can best be implemented through the use of a **clock**. If real clocks (or watches) are not available for each participant, it is possible to purchase small plastic non-working clocks or to make a substitute from paper plates, with movable cardboard hands attached with a paper fastener.

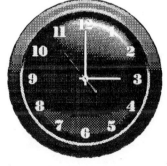

This would enable the resident to copy time from a real clock and to set the hands for mealtimes, activity beginnings and endings, etc. Time is a very important factor in activity planning. The following story points out the importance of reinforcing time in relation to routine with people who are confused.

*At one facility, the residents were accustomed
to having a group always come in before lunch
to present a bible study program. On one
occasion, because of scheduling difficulties, the
group came after lunch. When the program was
over, several of the residents asked to be taken
to lunch and refused to believe that they had
already eaten.*

Some of the more sophisticated means of using clocks are in
discussions of daylight savings time, time zones and what is
happening in other parts of the world at the same hour.

**Calendars**, too, can help with time orientation. Holidays,
birthdays (of both residents and famous people), events,
seasons, weather in relation to time of year, how many
days..., are all possible topics for activities and discussion.

*One inventive activities director[4] uses a reality
tree (a large branch covered with paper mache
and attached to a base) which the residents
decorate appropriately with homemade symbols.
Each month the tree looks different and the
decorations vary in degree of elaborateness.*

**Flowers** are nice to use and fun to smell. Each flower has a
season and often a time of day during which it releases its
greatest fragrance.[5]

- *Nicotiana* (Four O'Clocks) releases its fragrance
  after 4 pm.
- Petunia's scent is coarse until after dark.
- Lavender sold for its brighter hue of flowers
  smells of turpentine but the older, English

24

varieties (*Lavandula vera*) have duller flowers but brighter scents.
- Lilac hybrids which are newer with more showy flowers tend to have less scent then the old fashioned purple lilacs.

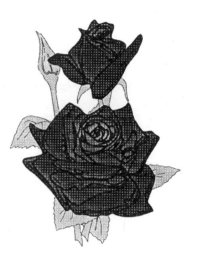

Matching pots of the same flower, matching a flower to the bottled scent of that flower or matching a pot of flowers to a picture of that kind of flower are all possible activities. If you are using bottled scents remember that the scents based in oil are better then those based in alcohol.

Orientation to place is also important and all types of **maps** can be helpful with this. The resident might be provided with a simple map of the facility with her/his room featured and the route s/he would take to meals and activities highlighted. Tours, using the map, would make it even more beneficial. Maps can be drawn to show field-trip locations and routes, the surrounding area, routes of parades that pass by, planned alterations and additions and almost any other thing that might be useful or interesting to depict. Actual maps can be utilized to pinpoint hometowns of residents, travel locations and other factual information. A game can be played in which a very large map is placed on the floor and residents are given beanbags to throw at it. The one who comes closest to the town in which the facility is located (or to his hometown) would be the winner.

The whole area of **food** suggests many possibilities for reality experiences. Menus, cookbooks, recipes and actual food can be used.

Activities can include:

— recipe swapping and comparing
— compilation of a cookbook
— food preparation and tasting

*One activities director[6] has had groups plan a dinner party for twenty-five guests, with each group of two or three being responsible for determining one course. The groups had no trouble with the meat (roast beef) or the dessert (ice cream with a variety of sauces), but those responsible for the potatoes couldn't agree and came up with four different kinds!*

*This idea was taken even further by another activities coordinator[7] who not only had a group plan a menu, but purchase the necessary food, prepare it and serve it. Of course, the limits were carefully set and much help and guidance was provided.*

**Photographs** are another valuable source of activity ideas. Not only can individuals' collections provide topics for discussion and reminiscing (and comparing!) but pictures taken at facility trips and celebrations can be used to remember people, locations and events. Photographs can, of course, be readily used to make scrapbooks, posters or collages and perhaps even used as a basis for contests. The question might be asked, "Do you recognize this scene?" or "How many of these occasions can you identify?"

**Newspapers** should not be overlooked as useful props, not only for current events, but discussions of food prices, contemporary fashions and feature articles. Several programs use the column "Dear Abby" as a discussion tool. A letter is read, the residents are asked to respond and then Abby's answer is read and compared.

The pictures on **cards** that were suggested in the section on matching activities can also be utilized in many other ways — picking favorites, selecting meals, comparing to actual objects are only a few of the possibilities.

*With a little imagination, unlikely household items can be utilized in reality activities. A particularly innovative geriatric specialist[8] uses an ordinary throw pillow which is passed around a group sitting in a circle. Questions are asked such as "What do you think it is stuffed with?", "Do you like the color?", "Do you like the shape?" Because there are no "right" answers and the leader is extremely supportive of their responses, participation is always good.*

*Similarly, she uses a large piece of interesting fabric, such as velvet tapestry in much the same manner. Everyone is invited to hold it while being asked questions — "What does it remind you of?" and "What would you like to do with it?" Residents often wrap themselves in it and respond with many different postures and answers.*

Many other articles would of course be used in much the same way with beneficial results.

# Music and Exercise

Music and exercise have been grouped together because it is difficult for most people to hear music without moving some part of their body. Indeed, music seems to affect many individuals who do not respond to other types of stimuli. And, it doesn't 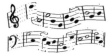 necessarily have to be the old-fashioned music exclusively; many people who are older respond well to rhythm of any kind — even disco!

**Music** has many purposes in activities programming. It is used to increase body movement and energy levels. It is useful for mood setting, relaxation and reminiscence and is commonly used with activities such as sing-alongs and rhythm band. Many other possibilities exist, including those that draw upon the resident's special capabilities.

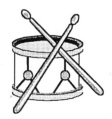 Games can be played with music, such as "Name That Tune", "Sing the next line", "What does the music make you think of?" and "Where were you when you first heard this song?" It is also possible to have people draw what music brings to mind.

*The previously mentioned specialist[9] uses music in many creative ways in her programs with older people. Using only their rhythm instruments, residents "talk" to each other.*

29

*Another variation is having each individual in turn come up with a rhythm that other group members repeat. Also they move to music, relying heavily on ethnic and lively melodies.*

*The success of her approach was borne out when a resident at another facility wandered into a staff demonstration. Although the leader was not familiar with the gentleman, she invited him to join in and participate with the group. He did so most willingly, demonstrating much enjoyment to the amazement of the staff members who knew him. Although he was obviously confused and had a reputation for non-participation, he was able to follow all instructions and become a full-fledged member of the group.*

**Dance** is also a source of possible activities, ranging from simply moving to music to wheelchair square-dancing. Many simple dance-type games and movements are very suitable for residents who are confused and disoriented. The wide variety of ethnic music available seems, in particular, to inspire motion, including the performance of remembered folk dances.

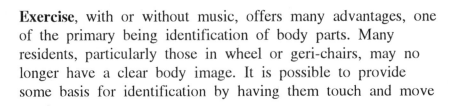

**Exercise**, with or without music, offers many advantages, one of the primary being identification of body parts. Many residents, particularly those in wheel or geri-chairs, may no longer have a clear body image. It is possible to provide some basis for identification by having them touch and move different parts of their bodies — with guidance and repetition of the names and locations of those parts. For safety, always start exercises with body parts below the waist. By starting exercises with the lower body you are decreasing the stress on the heart and reducing the chance of a heart problems during your activity.

Many different exercise programs have been devised for use with people who have disabilities or who are older. (See suggested reading list). The exercises given in **Safe Therapeutic Exercise for the Frail Elderly** by Hurley are effective and use simple, readily available materials such as sponge balls, sticks, towels and parachutes. Using these exercise activities, a full range of motion is given to all body parts with no part being overtaxed. Enjoyment and increased socialization also are benefits to those in exercise programs.

However, it is not necessary to present physical activity only as an exercise program (to which many people seem to have a natural resistance!). It can also be incorporated into other activities. Because it is very useful to wake people up and get their blood flowing before attempting to stimulate them mentally, simple body identification or rhythm exercises are often used as a preface to other reality activities. We are, after all, dealing with a total person, and it is difficult to effect change in one area, without affecting the rest of the person as well. Exercise need not — indeed, should not! —be difficult or strenuous, but just enough to wake people up and get them in tune with their bodies. Many of the simple games which will be outlined in the next section can also be used as forms of exercise.

31

# Games

Games offer a wide variety of different experiences for reality programming. Not only do they range from quiet to fairly active, from individual to large group but, of course, also from simple to increasingly complex. As with many other activities, often the same game can be modified to become increasingly more complex and challenging.

One game that can be used to illustrate this principle very well is **Wheel of Fortune**[10]. This is a simple board game involving a spinner and six pie-shaped wedges.

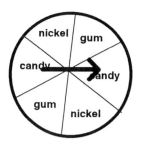

1 = nickel
2 = stick of gum
3 = candy

Initially, the resident spins and takes a prize from one of three numbered cups or bowls which the spinner indicates. After becoming familiar with the game, the symbols could be covered and the residents would have to identify their prizes by number only. Further modifications might be to add a "free choice" and/or "give one back" space. More complicated rules could also be added to determine the end and the winner of the game and the number of participants could be increased.

**Tic-Tac-Toe** is another concept that has many possible adaptations. A tic-tac-toe grid can be placed on the floor and two teams or individuals attempt to get three in a row, using two different colored beanbags. Another variation is to have individuals or teams involved in a guessing game; for each correct answer the resident gets the opportunity to place an O or X in a square until one side gets three in a row. **Modified Tic-Tac-Toe**[11] involves a board with nine symbols on it and a pack of 3x5 cards, each having one of the same symbols. The residents draw cards in turn, cover the matching symbol with a poker chip on the board until someone places three of their chips in a row. Flannel boards also lend themselves to this type of game and may be easier for some people to use than paper and pencil.

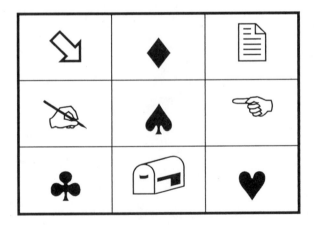

A **scavenger hunt** is another familiar game idea that can be utilized in many different ways. **Magazine scavenger hunts** are very popular for use with residents who are confused. A list of objects is provided; these items are then located in magazines and cut or torn out. There are many variations possible:

— individual or team activity
— pictures to match could be used instead of a list
— items could be a random selection or all related to one subject such as animals, transportation, Christmas or the season of the year
— the pictures could be collected into a scrapbook or collage when the game is completed

*For a regular scavenger hunt, one facility[12] distributed lists of things that were readily available to the residents — newspaper, greeting card, clothes hanger, pencil. They were requested to bring these items as admission to a party and the persons who brought the most articles on the list were awarded prizes.*

Another variation of this is to have the resident **feel objects that are concealed in a bag** and identify as many as possible, using only the sense of touch.[13] Similarly, **pictures of familiar items** (of the present or of the past) might be shown and the resident asked to guess what they are and/or what they are used for. This could also be done with **sound effect records** by asking "Guess what it is?" and "What else sounds like that?"

Many simple games can be played using materials that are inexpensive and readily available. Some ideas are:

- **ring toss** on the legs of a chair turned upside down on a table (jar rings or embroidery hoops can be used)
- **throwing pennies** into an aluminum pie pan that is floating in a tub of water
- **tossing clothes pins** into a plastic milk bottle (or a water pitcher or a laundry basket)
- **basketball toss** into a wastepaper basket, a smaller basket on a table or into a bottomless basket on an I-V pole
- **guessing games** — how many jelly beans in the jar, what's in the pillow, how many hearts in the picture?

**Holidays** provide many opportunities for games. The last mentioned game is a natural for many holidays, as are things such as tossing beanbags or "snowballs" (Styrofoam balls) at seasonal targets. **Word association games** can also be used — making words from the letters of the holiday or seeing how many other words can be thought of that are associated with the particular celebration. **Reminiscence** should also be encouraged, using questions such as "What was your all-time favorite Christmas present?" or "How did you celebrate the Fourth of July when you were a child?"

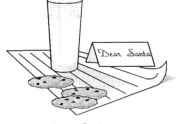

**Balls, balloons and beanbags** present numerous non-threatening opportunities for games. Some of these are **balloon volleyball, keeping a ball up in the air** on a parachute or sheet that is held by a group and **"catch"** with residents calling the names of other group members before throwing them the ball. An alternative might be to call residents by the color of the scarf that they are wearing.[14] (The scarves would be provided for each resident before the start of the game.)

Designing a **game based on orientation material** is another possibility. Simple statements could be written on 5x7 cards, such as Today is..., The season is..., The next meal is..., etc. An appropriate selection of answers could be placed on smaller 3x5 cards from which the players would select the correct answers. This could be done individually, in small groups or as a team effort.

**Matching games** are also very successful. Again the opportunities are endless. Go-together such as bread and butter, table and chair, pen and ink could be matched verbally, with pictures or with written words. Many of the ideas that were suggested in the section on matching could be incorporated into games and played with small groups.

# Crafts

Predicting the suitability of craft activities for residents who are confused is often difficult. Not only does performance vary because of confusion levels; but past skills, the degree of motivation and the amount of physical limitations and disabilities also have an effect. Experience has shown that some people are capable of doing complex craft projects while at the same time exhibiting high levels of confusion in other areas.

However, this discussion will be limited to group activities and those generally suitable for residents who are disoriented. Suggestions will be given in a broad, general sense, rather than with step-by-step directions which are readily available from other sources. If these, or any other, simple craft projects prove successful with a resident, it is then be possible to move on to something more complex — adding more steps, increasing colors used, offering choices.

One important aspect that should be stressed in planning a craft activity is that the finished product always has some recognizable use or purpose. If an individual is not able to complete a whole project, s/he should be shown a sample and told what his/her part will be in the finished product.

Some previously mentioned activities could also be used in a crafts program. For example, once **beads** have been sorted, they could be strung in a pattern of different colors or sizes — working from the simple to the more complex. It is helpful to provide a sample or the pattern worked out on paper, from which the resident could copy or match shapes and colors. Pictures that are selected in matching activities could be incorporated into **scrapbooks** and then given to children's groups or used in remotivation sessions. Indeed, scrapbooks make an excellent reality activity and can be structured to serve all kinds of purposes. One suggestion is to have each individual keep his/her own scrapbook of all those things that s/he likes or that have meaning for him/her. **Collages** can also be made using these same ideas.

Other simple craft techniques include:

— **crunch art** cutting tissue paper in small strips, crushing and gluing to fill in areas on large designs
— **paper mache** projects of all kinds
— **simple weaving** of baskets, pocketbooks, pot holders, etc., using short pieces of material (from which there are many to choose) and a limited number of colors to start
— **decorating** containers or boxes with shells or macaroni

**Pom-poms** provide a variety of possibilities, particularly with the looms that do not require winding through the middle of a closed circle. Many people can at least do part of the process, if not the final assembling. The same wrapping skills that are used in making pom-poms can also be used to cover various size cans with yarn to make wastebaskets or pencil holders.

**Ceramics** can also be utilized in a program of this type. Various materials that are available, such as play dough or salt dough might be explored as possible choices because they are less messy and, therefore, more desirable for some people to use. Some residents prefer only to decorate greenware, but many are capable of starting from scratch and creating useful, decorative ceramic pieces.

**Holidays** are a natural theme on which to base simple craft projects. In addition to the reality orientation tree previously mentioned, decorations, tray favors and corsages can be made utilizing a wide variety of suitable techniques. Recycled greeting cards can be made into puppets, baskets and Christmas tree ornaments by fairly simple procedures.

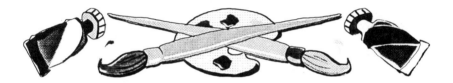

**Art media** should not be neglected. Finger painting, mural making, sketching and painting simple designs are all viable additions to an activities program for residents who are confused.

# Topics for Discussion

Discussion, both formal and informal, certainly plays a large role in reality activities. The following topics are just a few suggestions:

- Birthdays — birthplaces, zodiac signs, presents, memories
- Odors — (e.g. vanilla, pine, perfume) - What do they remind you of?
- Food — likes and dislikes, best meal eaten, food prices then and now, menu planning
- Trips — places visited, old autos in which rides were taken, things to take along

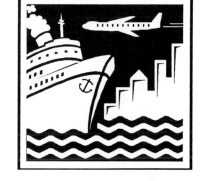

- Actors and actresses — films seen then and now
- Voting — politics, candidates, rallies, etc.
- School — memories, subjects studied, friends

The companion book to this one, **Activities for the Elderly Volume 2** by Parker and Will[15] has a set of discussion topics for each of its eighty plus activities. Exercising the resident's brain promotes increased circulation and stimulation. Encourage the resident to talk!

And, perhaps more importantly, every opportunity should be utilized to discuss things that occur in the facility — films, entertainment, meals, parties and everyday events.

# Selection of Activities

Although, as has been shown, many activity possibilities exist for use with residents who are confused and disoriented, the most difficult task often lies in selecting what is most suitable for an individual resident.

The most important factors in making this decision are:

1. the background information available on each individual
2. the specialized needs and goals that have been identified for each resident
3. the components of each activity — task breakdown

As always in activity selection, one starts with the resident and what is known about him/her. The background information should be reviewed and the resident's interests, educational level, life style and past experiences considered. Physical and cognitive limitations and capabilities must be included in this process.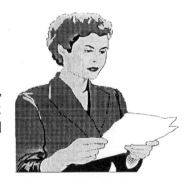

Building on this basic information, the next step is to precisely identify the resident's needs and goals. The more accurate the assessment, the easier it will be to select an activity which will satisfy him/her.

Some areas of need that are commonly found in residents who are confused and disoriented are for

Increased or improved
- self-esteem and confidence
- attention span
- social initiation
- social response
- social appropriateness
- appropriate response to stimuli
- orientation to person, place and/or time
- ability to find way around the facility (pathfinding skills)
- recognition of own name or those of others
- performance in self-help activities
- short-term memory function
- decision making ability
- adjustment to environment
- outlets for creative expression
- adjustment to disabilities or limitations

Decreased or reduced
- anxiety
- hostility
- suspicion
- fear of failure

It is essential to try to determine the specific needs of each individual; not just to group them together as the residents who are confused and disoriented. What are those things which seem to be a concern or interfere with his/her optimal functioning?

Does s/he get lost finding his/her way to the dining room? Does s/he forget where s/he is? Who s/he is? If s/he ate lunch yet? Does s/he confuse staff members with members of his/her family? Does s/he have a very low self-image? Is s/he unable to comb his/her own hair? To sit still and focus on a task for more than two or three minutes at a time? To choose what s/he wants to wear that day? To complete a simple game or project successfully?

Once some of these questions have been answered, it is easier to focus on what the projected outcome of an activity should be. It is important to remember that activity is only a means to an end, not the end itself!

Keeping this in mind then, the next step is to look at available activities and determine what might be applicable. Each part of the activity must be analyzed to determine its suitability. Some things to be considered are:

- Can it be done alone?
- What skills are necessary?
- Does it allow for a limited attention span?
- Can it be simplified?
- Could it be done by two persons or in a group?
- Is good eyesight, eye-hand coordination, stamina, balance, etc. required?
- Can familiar materials be used?
- Can success be assured?
- What assistance is necessary?
- How many steps must be remembered at one time?
- Are abstract concepts involved?

- Can immediate gratification or recognition be achieved?
- Can the skills learned be transferred to other activities?
- Are there many opportunities for error?
- Is judgment involved?
- Does it allow for socialization?

Once the appropriate activity or part of an activity has been selected, how it is presented to the resident also has great significance. How s/he is approached, the type of motivation provided, the environment, the teaching method and the quality and amount of time spent in instruction are all vital in determining success.

If the initial activity is well received and successfully performed, it is then possible to build on that success, one small step at a time, as previously described. It is important to remember that with most residents this will be a slow process, the initial steps perhaps requiring much time and patience. The more accurate the selection process, however, the better the chances are that progress ultimately will be achieved.

# Suggested Reading

Adil, J. 1994. **Accessible Gardening for People with Physical Disabilities: A Guide to Methods, Tools and Plants**. Bethesda, MD: Woodbine House.

Baratta-Lorton, M. 1972. **Workjobs**. Menlo Park, CA: Addison-Wesley Publishing.

Best Martini, E., M. A. Weeks and P. Wirth. 1994. **Long Term Care: Interpretation and Inspiration for Activity and Social Service Professionals**. Ravensdale, WA: Idyll Arbor, Inc.

Gordon, N. F. 1993. **Breathing Disorders: Your Complete Exercise Guide**. Champaign, IL: Human Kinetics Publications.

Hall, B. A. and M. M. Nolta. 1992. **The Activity Care Planning Cookbook: An "M.D.S." Based Guide to Building Better Resident Care Plans**. San Diego, CA: Recreation Therapy Consultants.

Helgeson, E.M. and Willis, S.C. 1987. **Handbook of Group Activities for Older Adults**. Binghamton, NY: The Haworth Press.

Hurley, O. 1988. **Safe Therapeutic Exercise for the Frail Elderly: An Introduction**. Albany, NY: The Center for the Study of Aging.

Nissenboim, S. and Vroman, C. 1989. **Interactions by Design: The Positive Interactions Program for Persons with Alzheimer's Disease and Related Disorders, Rev. Ed.** Omaha, NE: Geri-Active Consultants.

Parker, S. D. and C. Will. 1993. **Activities for the Elderly Volume 2: A Guide to Working with Residents with Significant Physical and Cognitive Disabilities**. Ravensdale, WA: Idyll Arbor, Inc.

Postiloff Fisher, P. 1995. **More than Movement For Fit to Frail Older Adults: Creative Activities for the Body, Mind and Spirit**. Baltimore, MD: Health Professions Press.

Sander, P. 1987. **Wake Up! A Sensory Stimulation Program for Nursing Home Residents.** La Grange, TX: M. & H. Publishing Company.

Sheridan, C. 1987. **Failure Free Activities for the Alzheimer's Patient**. Forest Knolls, CA: Elder Books.

Wessel, J.A. 1976. **I CAN Implementation Series**. Austin, TX: PRO-ED.

Wilder, L.B. 1974. **The Fragrant Garden: A Book About Sweet Scented Flowers and Leaves**. New York: Dover Publications, Inc.

Zgola, J.M. 1987. **Doing Things: A Guide to Programming Activities for Persons with Alzheimer's Disease and Related Disorders.** Baltimore, MD: Johns Hopkins Press.

# Footnotes

1    **Activities for the Elderly Volume 2** by Sandra D. Parker and Carol Will published by Idyll Arbor, Inc., P.O. Box 720, Ravensdale, WA 98051 (206) 432-3231.

2    Elizabeth L. Crepeau (1986). **Activity Programming for the Elderly.** Boston: Little, Brown and Company.

3    From Mary Baratta-Lorton in the book called **Workjobs** written in 1972 and published by Addison-Wesley Publishing Company, Menlo Park, CA.

4    Arlene Engle, Activities Director, South Cape Nursing Home, Cape May Court House, N.J.

5    For more information on floral scents please read **The Fragrant Garden** by Louise Beebe Wilder available through Dover Publications, 180 Varick Street, New York, NY 10014.

6    Dottie Plunkett, Activities Director (Retired), Friends Home, Woodstown, N.J.

7    Addie Simone, Activities Director, Shady Lane Home, Clarksboro, N.J.

8    Norma Goldberg, DTR, Registered Dance Therapist, Senior Clinical Instructor at Hahnemann Medical College, Philadelphia, PA

9    Norma Goldberg, DTR, Registered Dance Therapist, Senior Clinical Instructor at Hahnemann Medical College, Philadelphia, PA

10   Marie-France Boudreault, Vivien LaRue, and Lena Metzelaar, **To Live With Dignity** (Ann Arbor: The University of Michigan Press, 1975), p.19. Currently out of print.

11   **Concepts for Activity Coordinators** (Complimentary Issue), 1979

12   The Masonic Home and Charity Foundation, Burlington, N.J.

13   Dottie Plunkett, Activities Director (Retired), Friends Home, Woodstown, N.J.

14   Dottie Plunkett, Activities Director (Retired), Friends Home, Woodstown, N.J.

15   **Activities for the Elderly Volume 2** by Sandra D. Parker and Carol Will published by Idyll Arbor, Inc., P.O. Box 720, Ravensdale, WA 98051 (206) 432-3231.